THIS
MEMOIR JOURNAL
belongs to:

____

Are you ready to start writing your story?

This memoir journal has three sections:
- My early years
- Growing up fast (teen and adult life)
- About me now

Each left-hand page is for thinking,
then the right-hand page is for writing.

You can find extra space for longer stories
at the back of this book.

Write the stories that make your heart sing
and the stories that need to be told.

Start at page 1, or start wherever you like.
If a question does not apply, then change it.

Make this book your own!

My early years

Thinking about: my arrival

My name means: ______________________________

which is:

☐ a good description of me

☐ partly true

☐ not really me at all

My star sign is: ______________________________

so I'm supposed to be:

____

which I think is:

☐ quite accurate

☐ possibly true

☐ nothing like me!

My name

1

I was born on: ________________________________

and given the name: ________________________________

____

I was given this name because: ________________________________

____

____

Over the years I've had nicknames like: ________________________________

____

____

____

Now I prefer to be called: ________________________________

____

____

Thinking about: my family

This stick-figure drawing or copy of an old photo shows my family (or the people I lived with).

As a baby...

I was born in: _______________________________

____

____

____

I grew up with my: _______________________________

____

____

____

There were _______ people in my family: _______________

____

____

____

I'd describe our home as: _______________________________

____

____

Thinking about: the mini-me

What people said about me…

☐ Good as gold…

☐ A bit of a handful…

☐ Full of beans…

☐ In another world…

☐ Sharp as a tack…

☐ ___________________

Best toy as a toddler:

Best toy as a pre-schooler:

When I was small

People described me as: _________________

____

____

____

Looking back, I'd describe myself as: _________________

____

____

____

I was happiest when I was: _________________

____

____

____

The toys and games I loved most were: _________________

____

____

Thinking about: family and culture

Words that describe my family (or people I lived with):

- ○ close-knit
- ○ reserved
- ○ loud
- ○ traditional
- ○ wild
- ○ funny
- ○ devout
- ○ quirky
- ○ ______________________
- ○ ______________________

Things we did that made us special:

____

____

My background 

At home, we spoke: ______________________________

For me, English was: ______________________________

My family originally came from: ______________________________

The holidays we celebrated were: ______________________________

Thinking about: key people

The key people in my early life were:

_________________ , who was my _________________

_________________ , who was my _________________

_________________ , who was my _________________

_________________ , who was my _________________

_________________ , who was my _________________

_________________ , who was my _________________

_________________ , who was my _________________

_________________ , who was my _________________

_________________ , who was my _________________

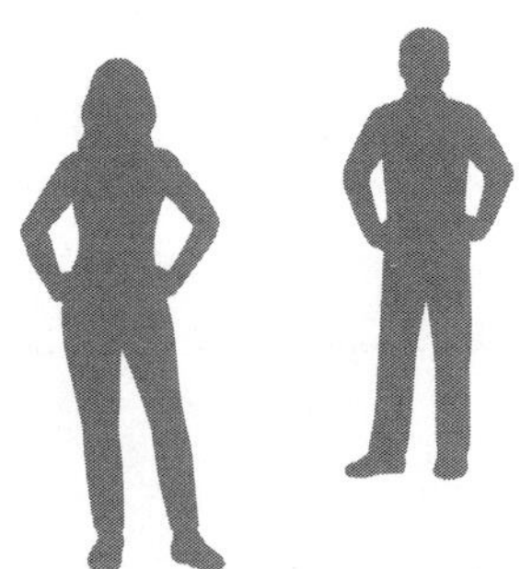

People around me

As a child, I spent most of my time with: ___________________

____

____

____

My relatives were: ___________________

____

____

____

The people living nearby were: ___________________

____

____

____

I really loved: ___________________

____

____

____

Thinking about: early school life

Best teacher: _______________________

Best friend: _______________________

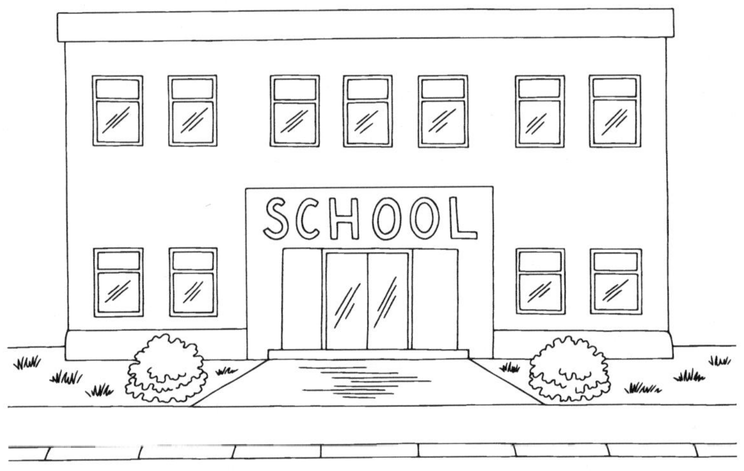

Actually, my school looked more like this:

Starting school

When I started school, I felt: _______________________

____

____

____

My teachers were: _______________________

____

____

____

In class, I liked: _______________________

____

____

____

In the playground, I always: _______________________

____

____

Thinking about: my activities

- ☐ Every sport I could
- ☐ Indoor activities only
- ☐ Garage pingpong
- ☐ Climbing trees
- ☐ Elastics / French skipping
- ☐ Bike-riding
- ☐ Dancing
- ☐ Athletics
- ☐ Trampolining
- ☐ At the pool (deep or shallow?)
- ☐ Side wall tennis
- ☐ Back street soccer
- ☐ Team captain
- ☐ __________________________
- ☐ __________________________

Any awards, prizes, trophies?

Getting active

I loved watching: _______________

I loved playing: _______________

I was good at: _______________

I always wanted to: _______________

Thinking about: the rules at home

The rules were:

- [ ] Relaxed
- [ ] A bit strict
- [ ] The same as for most kids
- [ ] Super strict

I got into trouble for:

- [ ] Answering back
- [ ] Being late
- [ ] Squabbling
- [ ] Forgetting things

I was actually good at:

- [ ] Looking after the little ones
- [ ] Being organised
- [ ] Being polite to adults
- [ ] Helping at home

In THIS house, we...

The rules at home were: _______________________

____

____

____

The unspoken rules were: _______________________

____

____

____

I got into trouble when I: _______________________

____

____

____

Looking back, I: _______________________

____

____

Thinking about: my best ever

Best ever gift:

Best ever event:

Best ever gift I made:

Best ever surprise:

Best ever treat:

Special days

At weekends, we often: _______________

On my birthday: _______________

On special holidays or parties: _______________

My best ever present was: _______________

Thinking about: my chores

My chores were:

- ◯ Farm or yard work
- ◯ Housework
- ◯ Feeding animals
- ◯ Washing dishes
- ◯ Nothing at all
- ◯ _______________________

When I was free, I would:

- ◯ Hang out with friends
- ◯ Race from activity to activity
- ◯ Stay in my room
- ◯ _______________________

Chores and fun

My chores at home were: _______________

____

____

Pocket money was: _______________

____

____

When I had free time, I: _______________

____

____

My idea of fun was to: _______________

____

____

Thinking about: places we went

Places we went for the day:

- ☐ The pool
- ☐ The library
- ☐ National parks
- ☐ Sports events
- ☐ The beach
- ☐ _______________________

Places we went for longer:

- ☐ Relatives' houses
- ☐ Camp sites
- ☐ Holiday parks
- ☐ Motels
- ☐ Hotels
- ☐ _______________________

Time out!

In school holidays or summer break, we often: _______

____

____

____

If we went away, we: _______________________________

____

____

A 'big trip' meant: _________________________________

____

____

My travel dream was to: _____________________________

____

____

Thinking about: meals back then

Typical breakfast:

Typical snacks:

Typical lunch:

Typical evening meal:

Typical special treats:

Glorious food

At home, cooking was done by: ________________

____

____

____

The food I loved most was: ____________________

____

____

____

We had fast food when: ________________________

____

____

____

I learned to cook: ____________________________

____

____

____

Thinking about: life at home

- [ ] Urban
- [ ] Suburbs
- [ ] Countryside
- [ ] ___________________________

- [ ] One house for my whole childhood
- [ ] A few houses
- [ ] On the move all the time
- [ ] ___________________________

- [ ] My own bedroom AND play area
- [ ] My own bedroom
- [ ] Are you kidding? Shared bedroom!
- [ ] ___________________________

- [ ] Big back yard
- [ ] Played in the street
- [ ] Balcony only
- [ ] ___________________________

At home

We lived in a: _______________

____

____

____

Most of my friends lived in: _______________

____

____

____

My bedroom or personal space was: _______________

____

____

____

I liked to hang out in: _______________

____

____

Thinking about: animals

As a child, I loved:

○ cats

○ dogs

○ birds

○ _______________________________

If I went to a zoo or nature park, I rushed to see
the: _______________________________
and the: _______________________________

If I had a spirit animal, it would have been a:

____

Pets and animals

As a child, I loved: _______________________

____

____

____

For me, pets were: _________________________

____

____

____

I always wished I could have a: ____________

____

____

____

I often think about: _______________________

____

____

____

Thinking about: my growing-up self

As I grew up, I became more:

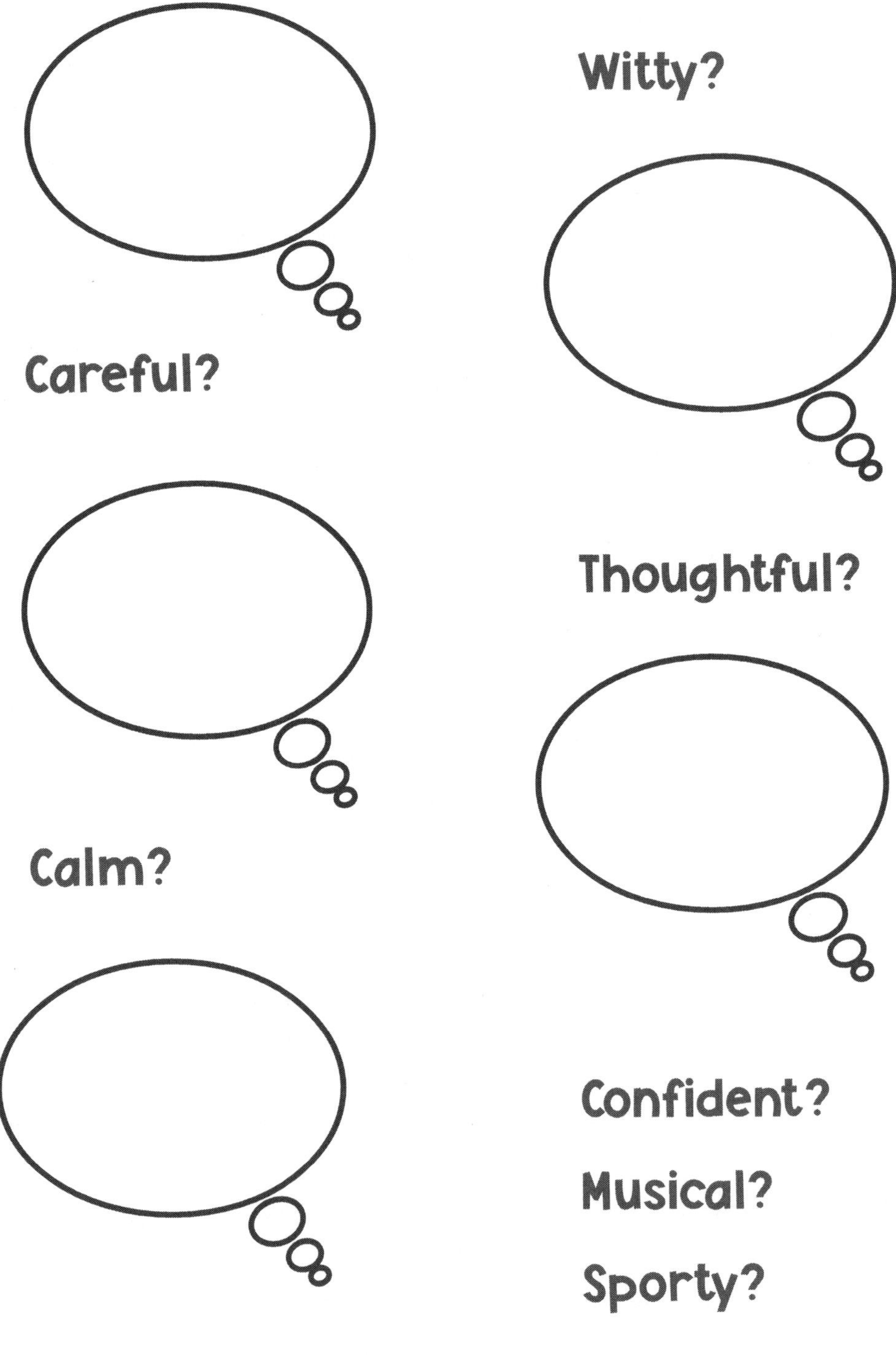

My strengths

I was keen to learn: _______________________

____

____

____

With people, I could always: ________________

____

____

____

I was creative with: _______________________

____

____

____

I still laugh about how I: ___________________

____

____

More about my childhood

Growing up fast

Thinking about: high school days

Teachers or students that made an impact on me:

Name (or description)	Reason

My student self

My high school teachers were: _______________

____

____

____

My attitude was mostly: _______________

____

____

____

The subjects I liked best were: _______________

____

____

____

I wanted to be a: _______________

____

____

____

Thinking about: time out of school

Typical things I'd do:

- ☐ Cycle around
- ☐ Go to the pool or beach
- ☐ Catch a bus to meet up with friends
- ☐ Meet at the basketball or tennis courts
- ☐ Go hiking
- ☐ Play with a team
- ☐ Play with several teams
- ☐ Play in championships
- ☐ _______________________
- ☐ _______________________
- ☐ _______________________

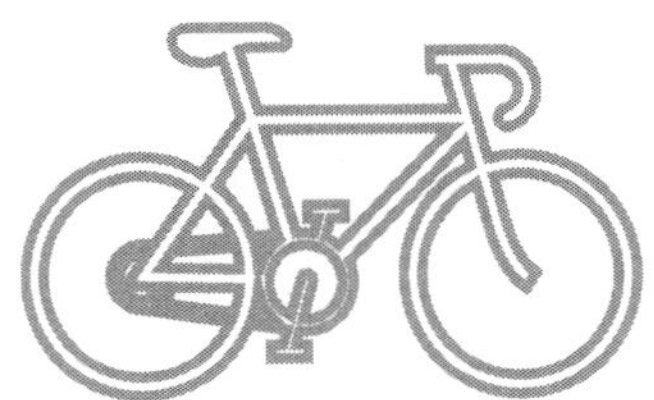

Sport and exercise... ⑰

Getting outdoors meant: _______________________

____

____

____

The sport and exercise I liked most: _____________

____

____

____

I was best at: ___________________________________

____

____

____

I always wanted to: ______________________________

____

____

Thinking about: more best ever...

Best ever family outing:

Best ever place to hang out with friends:

Best ever group of friends:

Best ever special event:

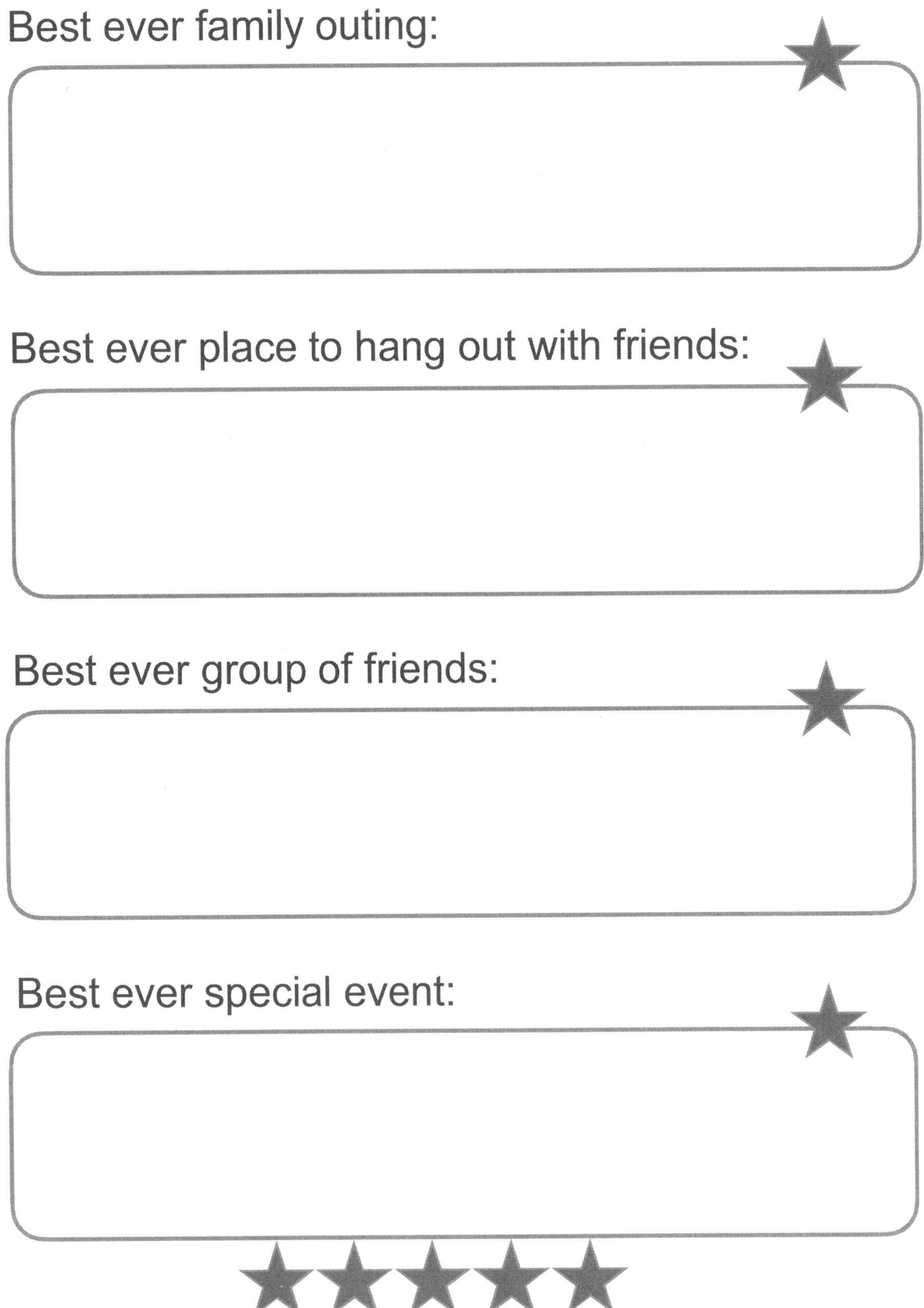

Good times, fun times

At home, as a family, we: ______________________

____

____

____

With my friends, I: ______________________

____

____

____

I was allowed out with: ______________________

____

____

____

I had to be home by: ______________________

____

____

____

Thinking about: what I loved

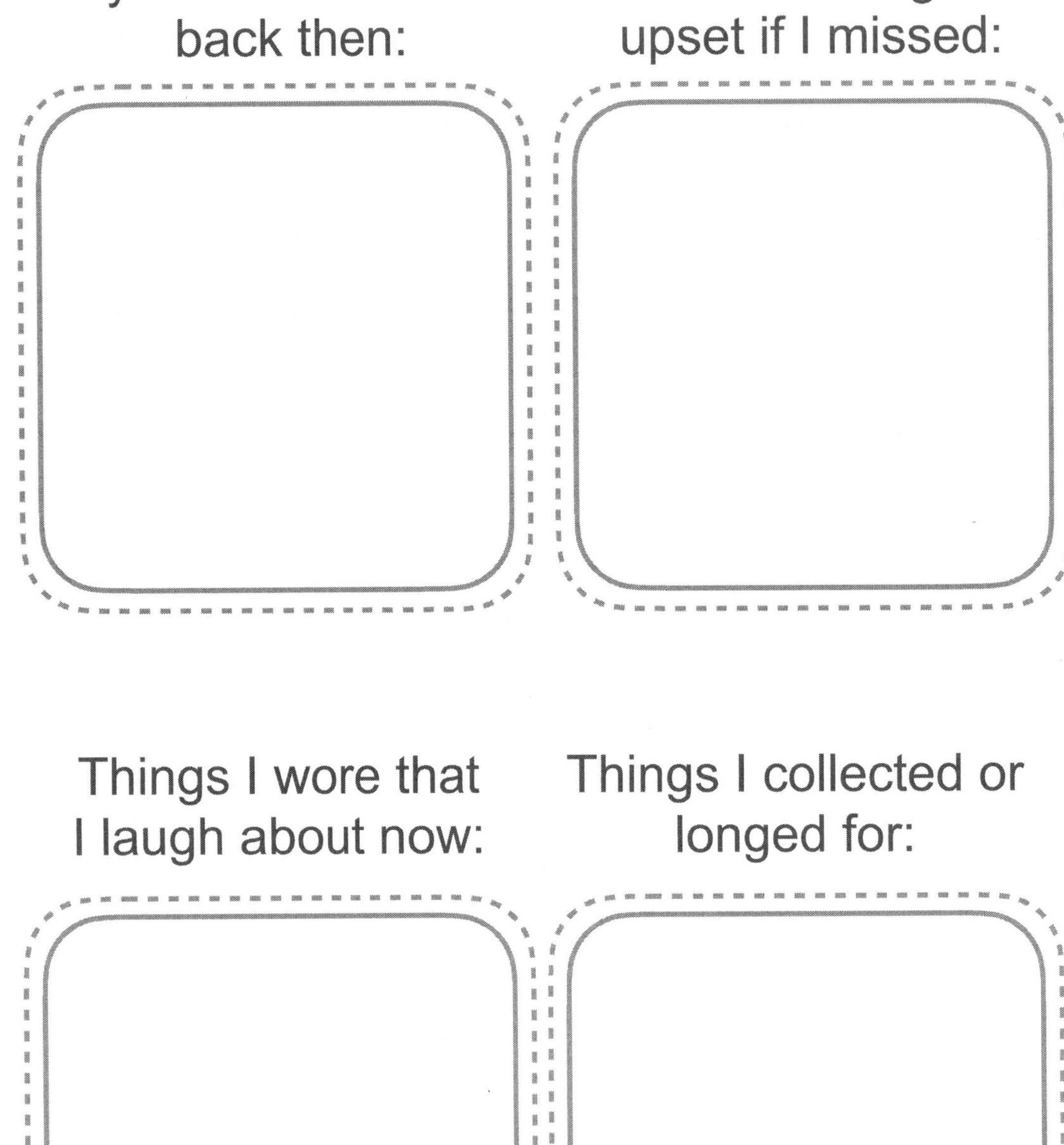

Back in the day...

I enjoyed music like: ______________________

____

____

____

I enjoyed TV shows like: ______________________

____

____

____

I enjoyed movies like: ______________________

____

____

____

I wore clothes like: ______________________

____

____

Thinking about: the old days

Things that kids today will never know:

- Going to the video store

- Making compilation cassette tapes

- Texting on the first mobile phones

- The sound of dial-up internet

- One landline phone at home

- Massive encyclopedia sets

- No seat belts in the back of the car

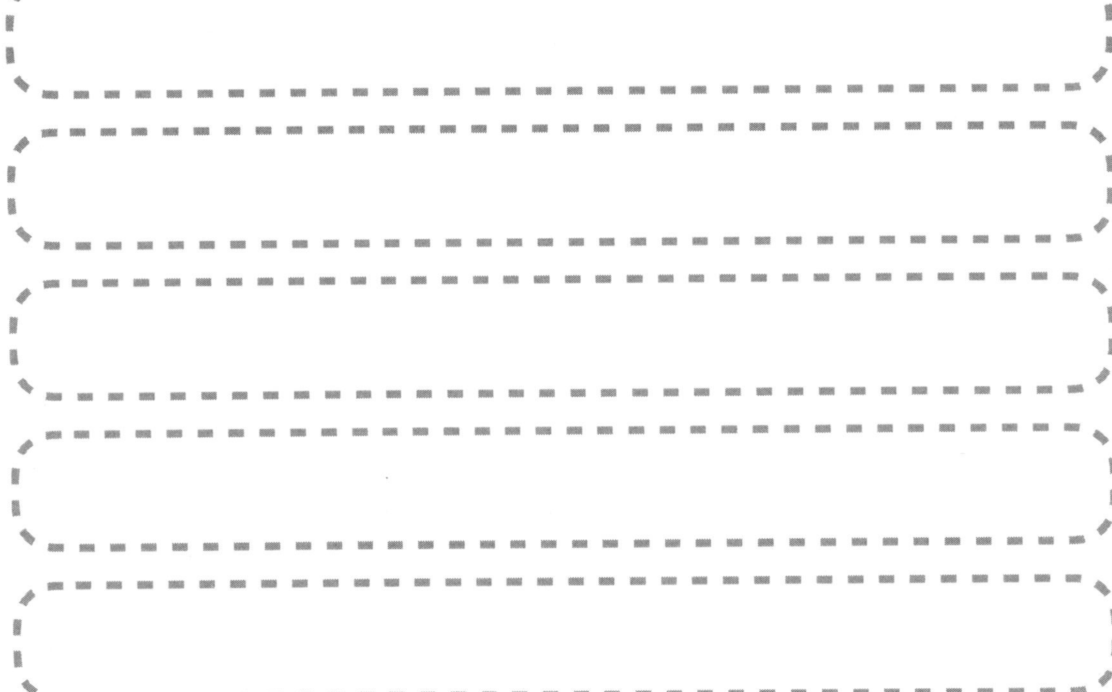

A changing world 

We NEVER had: _______________________

____

____

____

'Technology' meant: _______________________

____

____

____

In those days, kids: _______________________

____

____

____

It was good that we: _______________________

____

____

____

Thinking about: my dating story

- ◯ Secretly dating
- ◯ Visibly dating
- ◯ Not dating at all!

- ◯ Conventional
- ◯ On my own terms

- ◯ Confident
- ◯ Anxious?

- ◯ Being my real self
- ◯ Feeling I had to fulfil a role

- ◯ Earlier than friends
- ◯ Later than friends

- ◯ In love
- ◯ More like best friends

Someone special?

'Dating' was:

I thought that:

My parents thought that:

Eventually, I:

Thinking about: my pathway

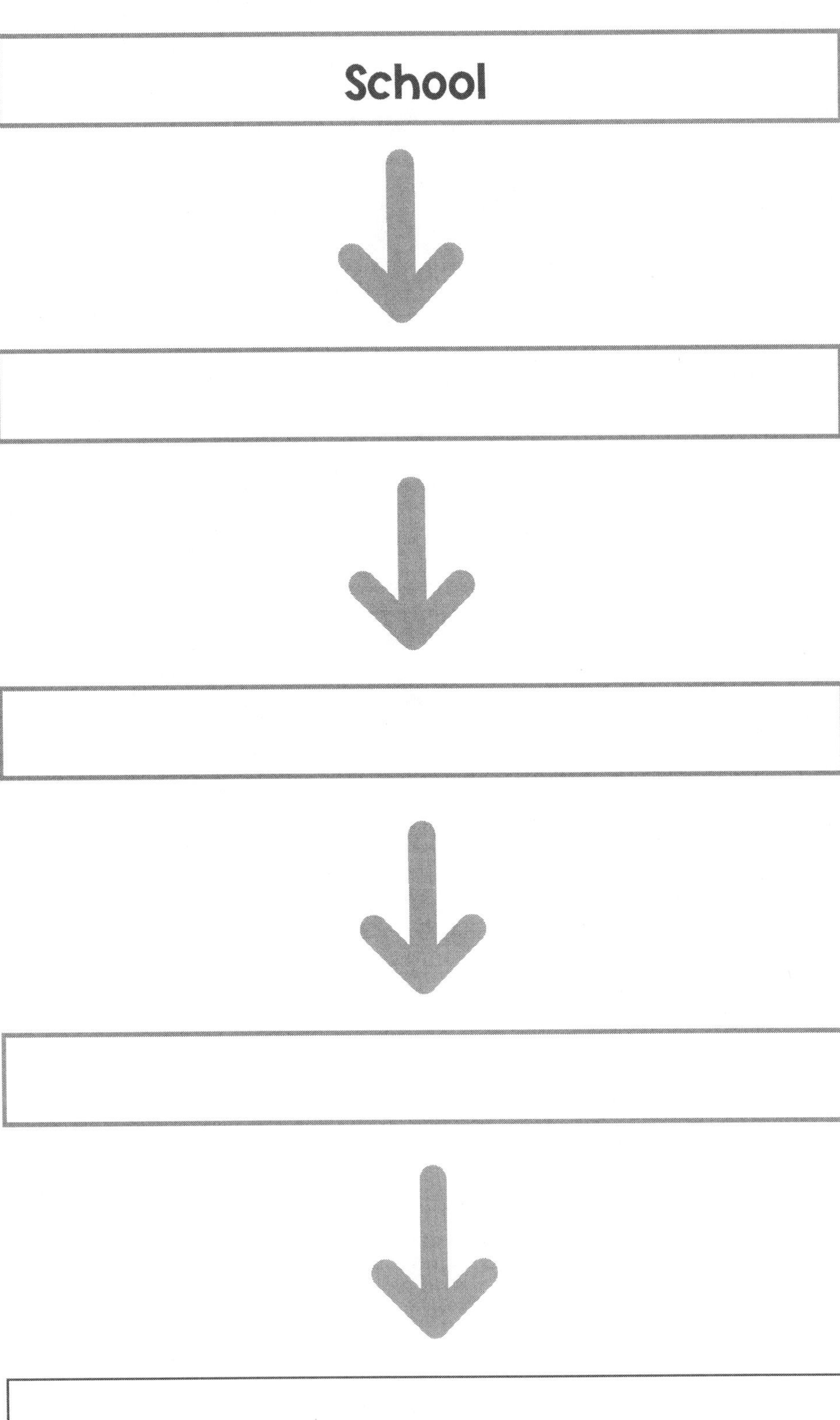

Next steps

Leaving school meant: _______________

I celebrated by: _______________

My next step was: _______________

After that, I: _______________

Thinking about: first paid work

- [ ] babysitting
- [ ] gardening
- [ ] dog walking

- [ ] serving food
- [ ] kitchen work
- [ ] paper delivery

- [ ] building, digging
- [ ] farm hand
- [ ] fruit picking

- [ ] store assistant
- [ ] check-out staff
- [ ] factory work

- [ ] coaching
- [ ] tutoring
- [ ] office work

My first paid work was at age: ___

My first full-time job was at age: ___

ALSO unpaid work:
- [ ] volunteering
- [ ] caring
- [ ] family business

Hard at work!

My first paid job was: _______________________

____

____

My first full-time job was: _______________________

____

____

I learned a lot from: _______________________

____

____

I contributed a lot to: _______________________

____

____

Thinking about: transport

I know how to ride/drive a:

- ◯ bike
- ◯ motorbike
- ◯ car
- ◯ motorhome
- ◯ truck or lorry
- ◯ boat
- ◯ plane
- ◯ skateboard
- ◯ horse

◯ _______________
◯ _______________
◯ _______________

I have travelled by:

- ◯ cruise ship
- ◯ jet ski
- ◯ helicopter
- ◯ camel
- ◯ tram or streetcar
- ◯ cable car

◯ _______________
◯ _______________
◯ _______________

Getting around

I mostly got around by: _______________________

____

____

Learning to drive was: _______________________

____

____

For me, the best way to travel: _______________

____

____

In my dreams, I: _____________________________

____

____

Thinking about: interactions

I'd describe myself then as:

☐ Always a leader
☐ Great team player
☐ More of a loner

☐ Upbeat
☐ Sometimes moody
☐ A joker

☐ Needing people
☐ Needing people AND solitude
☐ Needing time to think

☐ Obsessional
☐ Laid-back
☐ Short-tempered

☐ Indoor person
☐ Outdoor person
☐ Both, really

☐ Always first
☐ Whatever…
☐ Last on principle!

☐ Leaping into action
☐ Thinking things through
☐ Needing a push

Getting together

My interests as I got older were: ________________

____

____

____

I connected with groups like: ___________________

____

____

____

It was good when: _____________________________

____

____

____

I've never lost my passion for: __________________

____

____

____

Thinking about: key events for me

FALL OF BERLIN WALL!

        TITANIC WRECKAGE DISCOVERED!

WALL STREET CRASH!

        ROYAL WEDDING!

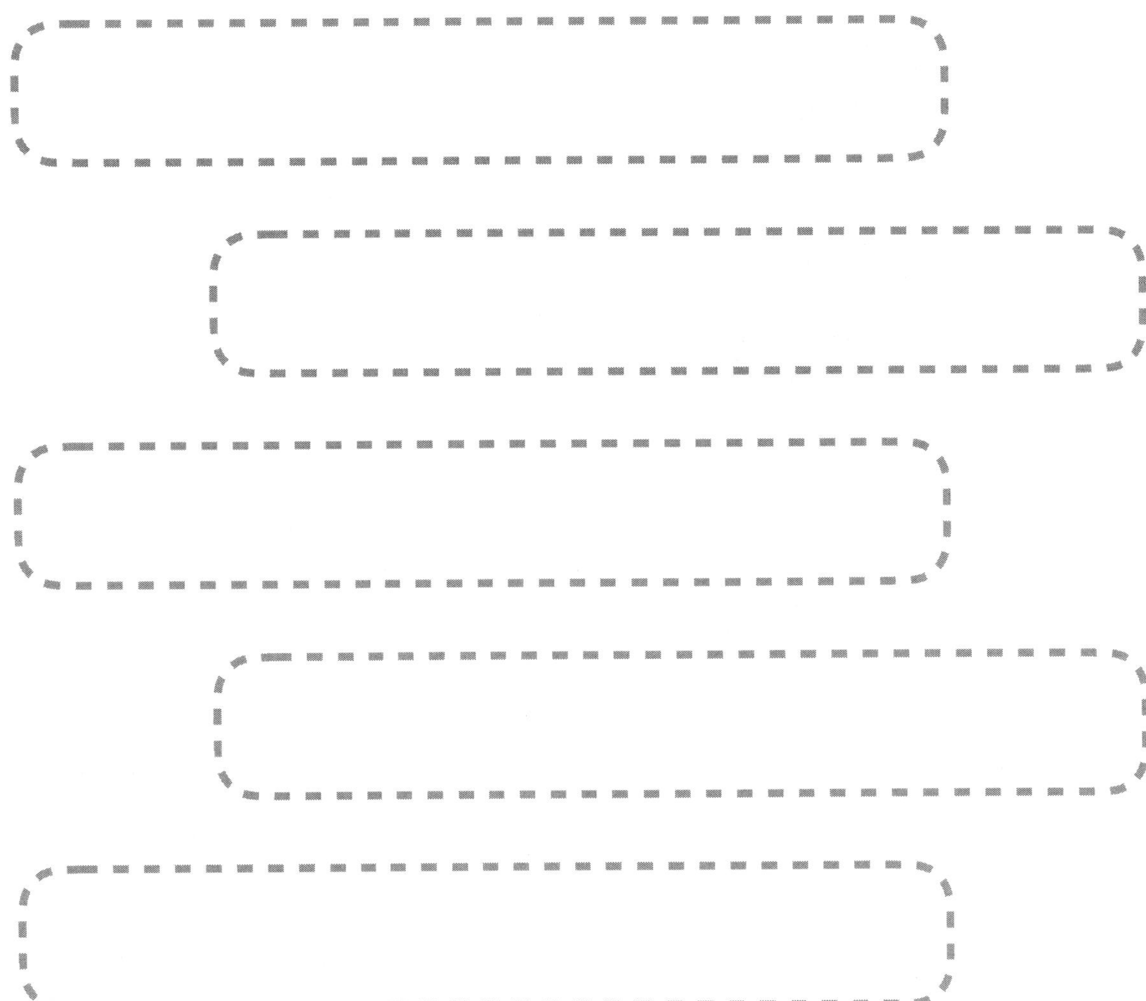

Living through history (26)

World events I've lived through: _______________________

Ways I've been involved: ______________________________

Things that changed my life: __________________________

Small ways I've made a difference: ____________________

Thinking about: the loves of my life

People? Pets? Cars? Projects?

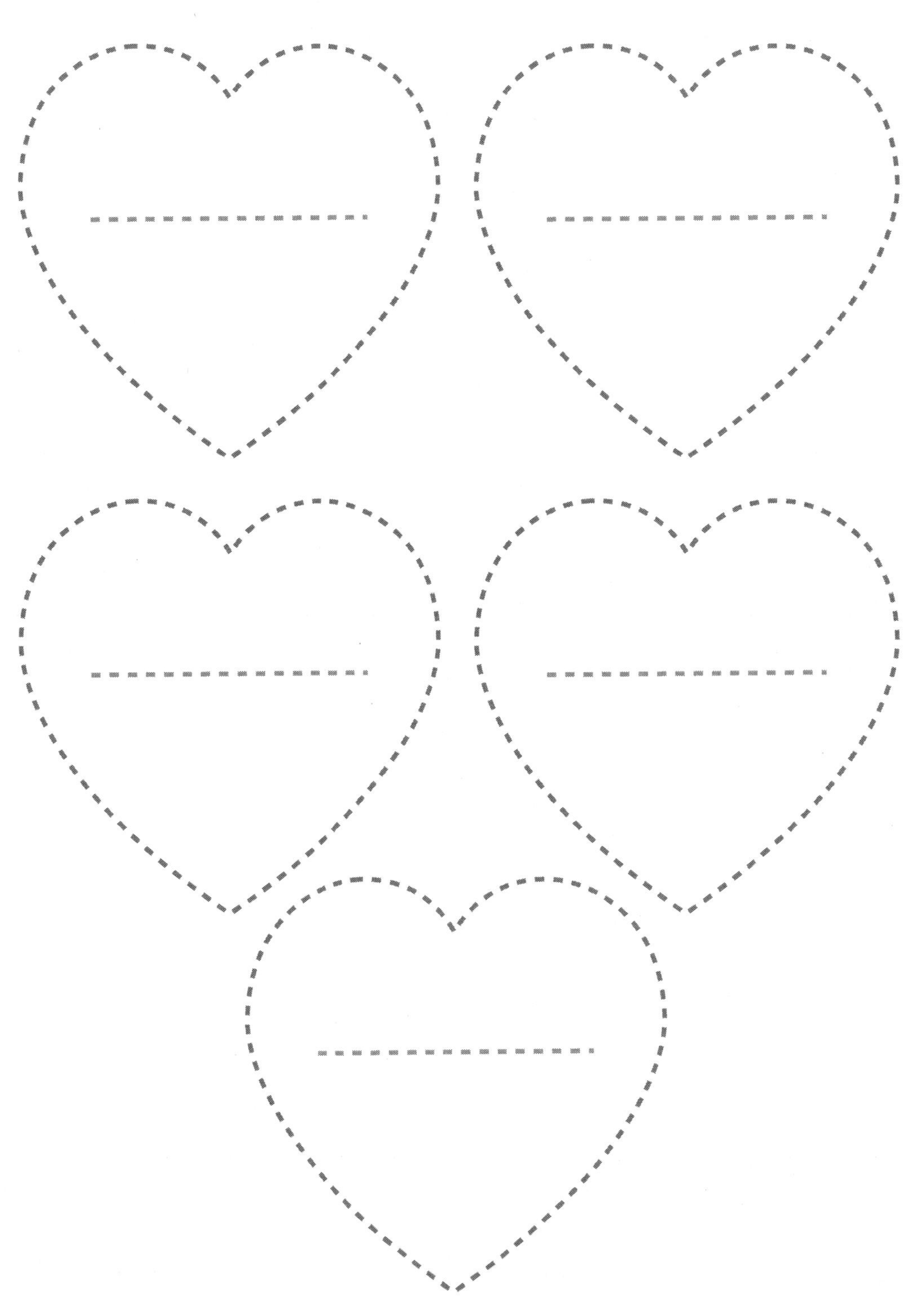

Love, love, love?

27

My relationships have been: _______________________

____

____

____

I'm grateful for: _______________________

____

____

____

I wish that: _______________________

____

____

____

Right now I really appreciate: _______________________

____

____

Thinking about: places and homes

Places I've lived:

____

____

____

Homes I've lived in:

____

____

____

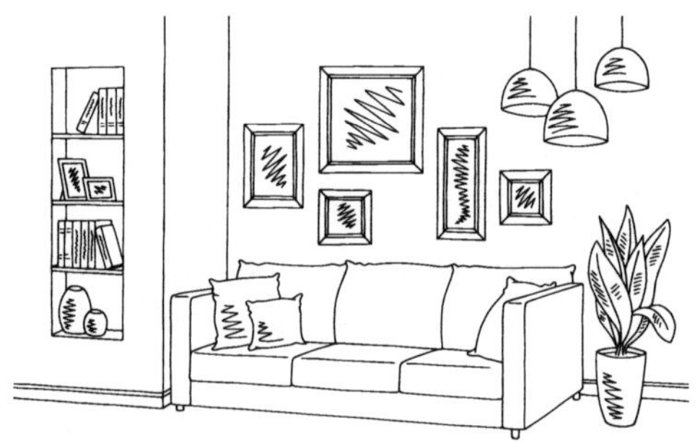

House and garden

28

I moved out of the family home when: ______________

____

____

____

I liked living in: ______________________

____

____

____

I spent a lot of time working on: ______________

____

____

____

I was proud of my: ____________________

____

____

____

Thinking about: who I've been

☐ A parent or step-parent to:

☐ An aunt or uncle to:

☐ A friend or mentor to:

☐ A grandparent to:

Children in my life

The names of the children in my life: ___________

And they are my: ___________

What I've learned from kids: ___________

What they've given me: ___________

Thinking about: awards

Awards or praise I've received
(or awards I should have had!)

for: _______________________

for: _______________________

for: _______________________

for: _______________________

All my roles

Different roles I've had in my life are: ________________

I feel good about my: ________________

The best work I've done is: ________________

My greatest achievement has been: ________________

More about growing up

About me now

Thinking about: my impact

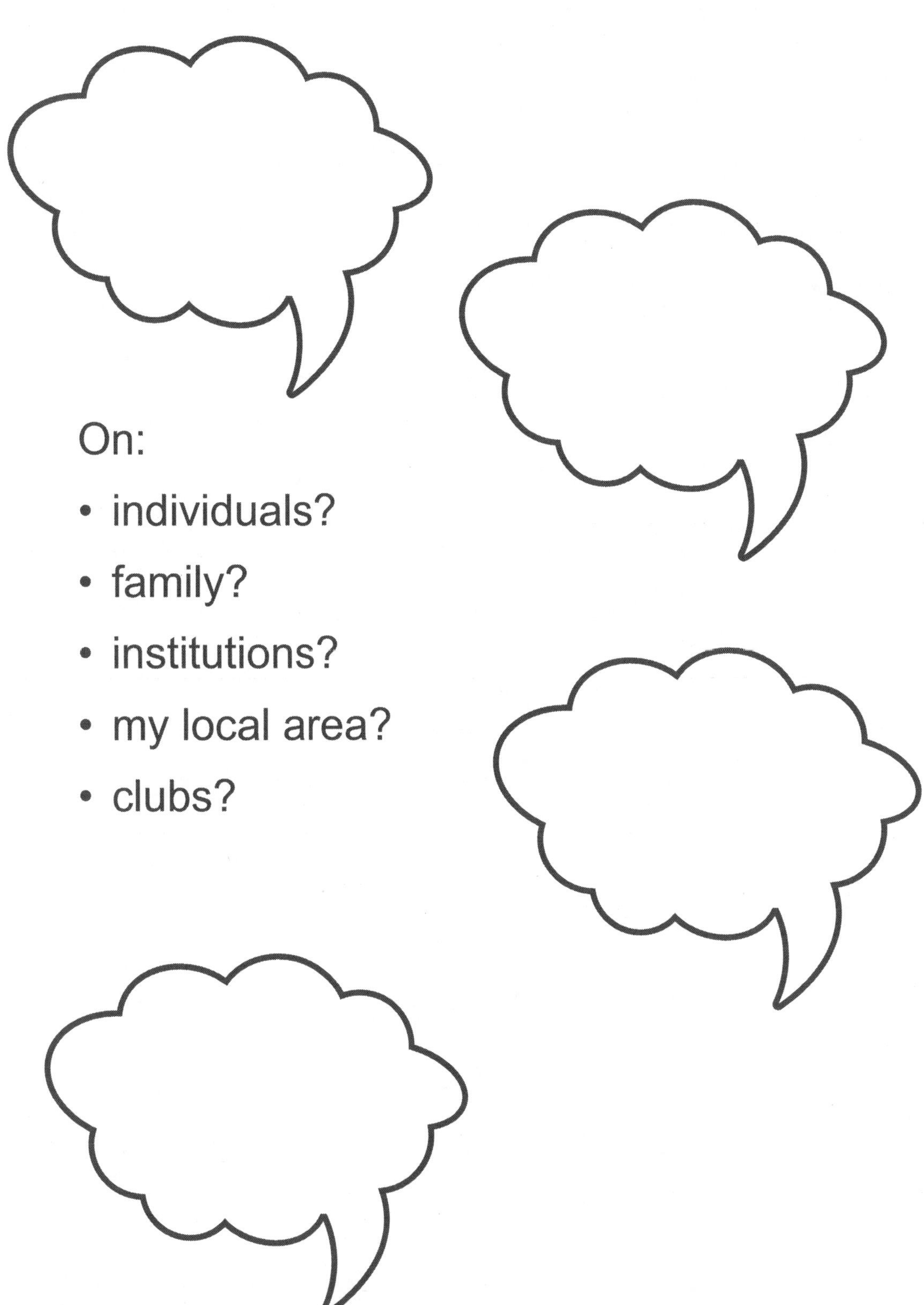

On:

- individuals?

- family?

- institutions?

- my local area?

- clubs?

The legend...so far

I know I've made an impact on: _______________________

____

____

I'm proud to say I: _______________________________

____

____

People talk about how I: ___________________________

____

____

My goals now are: ________________________________

____

____

Thinking about: where I've been

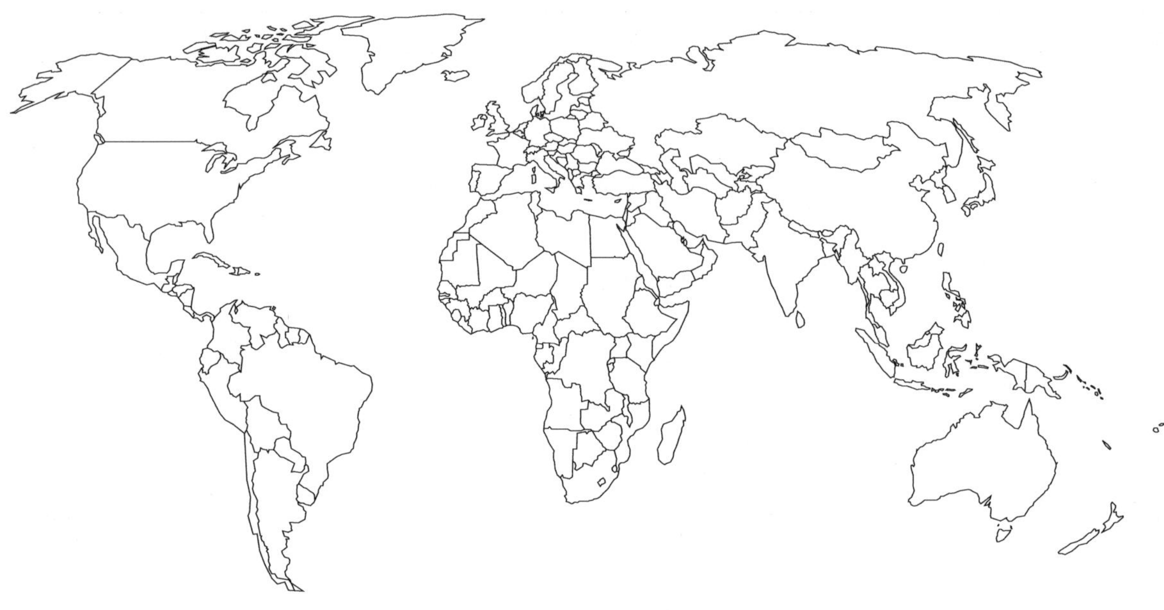

Where have you lived or visited?
Around the world or closer to home?

Places and adventures (32)

An outstanding event in my life: ______________________

____

____

A famous person I met: ________________________________

____

____

An amazing travel experience was: ______________________

____

____

A real adventure was: _________________________________

____

____

Thinking about: people I admire

These are the awards I'd give:

To:

for:

To:

for:

To:

for:

To:

for:

People that mean a lot (33)

The most important people in my life are: ___________

It's great to catch up with: ___________

I love it when I hear from: ___________

I want to reconnect with: ___________

Thinking about: my creative self

Artist?

Builder?

Inventor?

Musician, singer?

Composer?

Cook?

Crafter, woodworker?

Dancer?

Garden designer?

Party planner?

Writer?

Poet?

Photographer?

Programmer?

Entrepreneur?

Organiser?

Problem solver?

Builder?

Team builder?

Fixer of broken-down goods?

Fixer of broken-down dreams?

Making and creating 

Projects I've enjoyed: _______________________

____

____

____

I've been told I have a gift for: _______________________

____

____

____

Now I want to focus on: _______________________

____

____

____

I'd love to: _______________________

____

____

____

Thinking about: groups in my life

Groups I've been part of:

Groups I'm still part of:

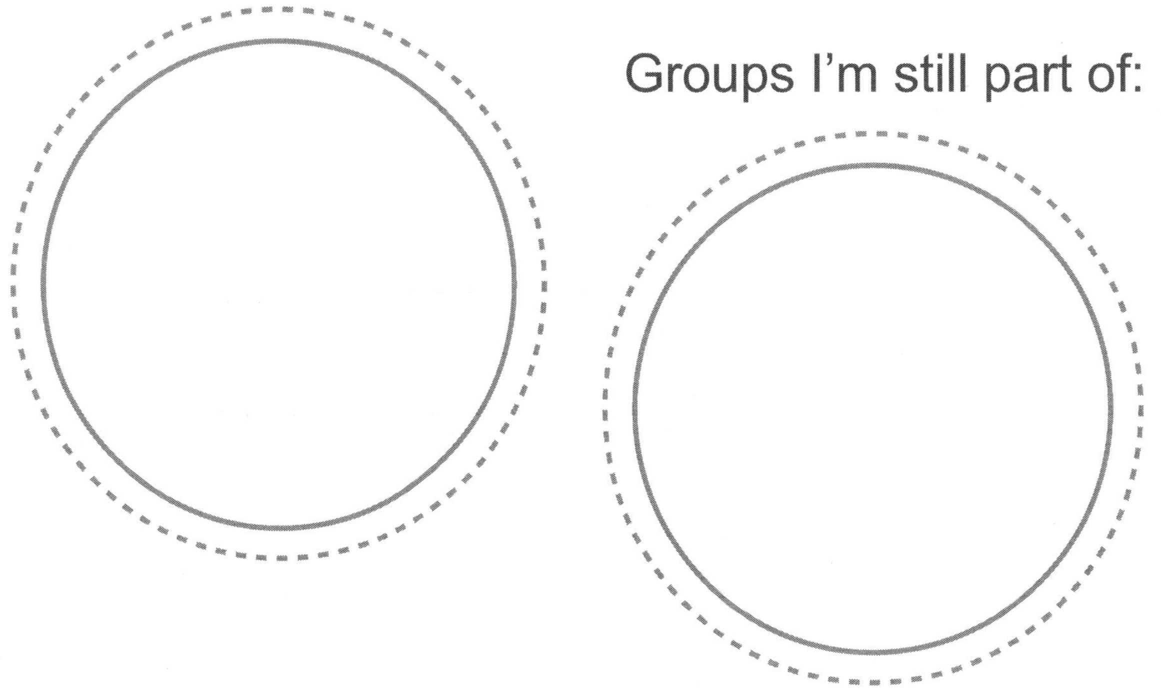

Recommended, haven't got there yet:

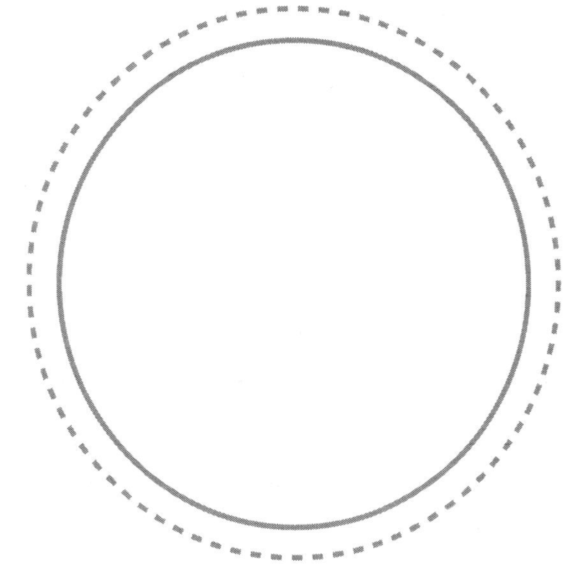

Online?

In person?

Not a group person?

Active and connected

For me, getting outdoors is: _______________________

____

____

I like to keep active by: _______________________

____

____

Groups that give me energy: _______________________

____

____

Trying new things is: _______________________

____

____

Thinking about: who will listen?

These are the people who said

'Call or message me any time.'

(A ticked box shows the number is in my phone.)

In conversation... (36)

I like to talk about: _______________________

____

____

I know a lot about: _______________________

____

____

I want my voice to be heard about: _______________________

____

____

It's not always easy, but I: _______________________

____

____

Thinking about: music and me

Music that changes my mood:

Music that speaks to my soul:

Music I just can't get into:

Music that takes me back:

My 'Desert Island' picks

Three songs (or albums): _______________________

____

____

____

Three 'best ever' movies: _______________________

____

____

____

Three books I'd take to that desert island: _________

____

____

____

Three photo collections: _______________________

____

____

____

Thinking about: in the perfect world

I'd love to have met:

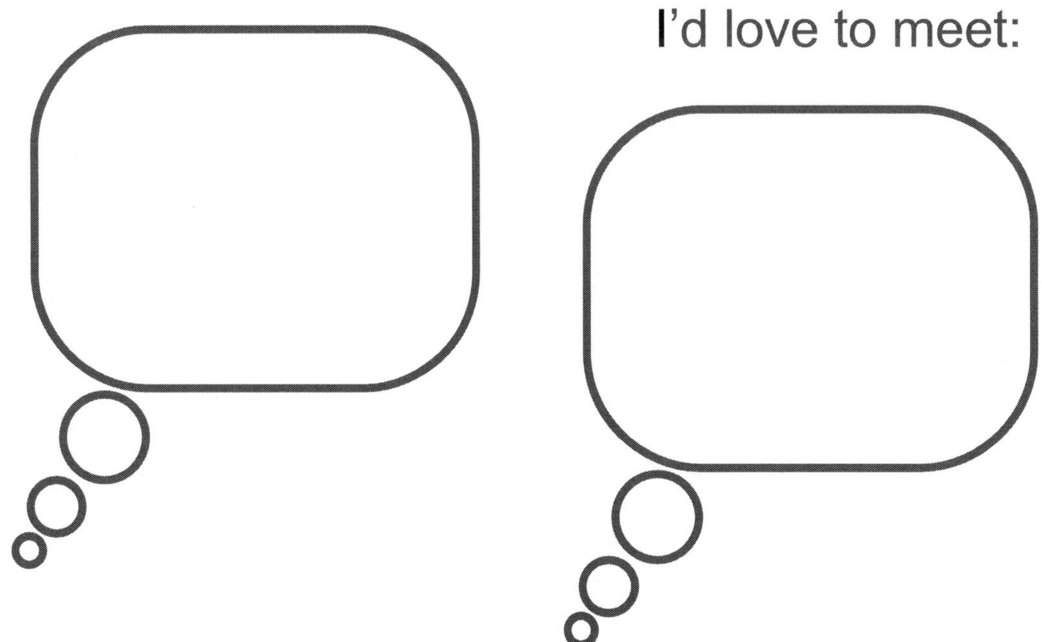

I'd love to meet:

I'd love to have seen:

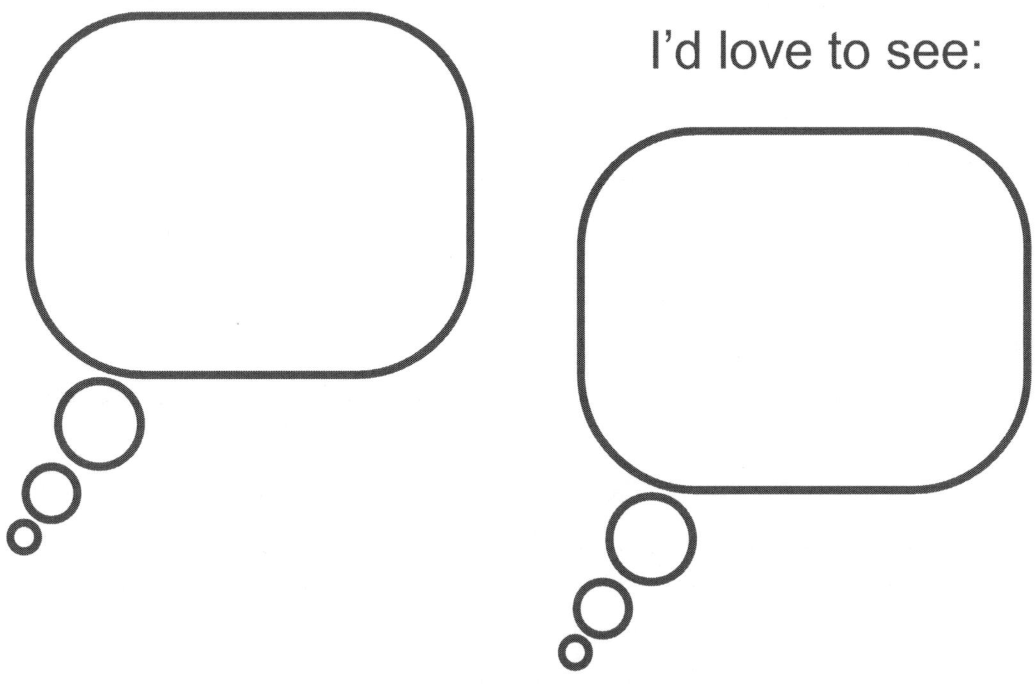

I'd love to see:

My dream event

My perfect event or meal would be: _______________

____

____

____

In the perfect location of: _______________

____

____

____

With my companions: _______________

____

____

____

And we'd talk about: _______________

____

____

____

Thinking about: what helps?

What helps, on a not-so-good day?

☐ Talking about it OR
☐ Working through it myself?

☐ Getting a hug OR
☐ Going for a walk?

☐ Calling a friend OR
☐ Meeting with a group?

☐ Getting lost in activity OR
☐ Sitting quietly in nature?

☐ Listening to music OR
☐ Having peace and quiet?

☐ Doing something new OR
☐ Doing something familiar?

I'm at my best when I: _______________________

____

____

____

I know I can get support from: _______________

____

____

____

I can be kind to myself when I: _______________

____

____

____

I've had to redefine my idea of: _______________

____

____

____

Thinking about: what I prefer

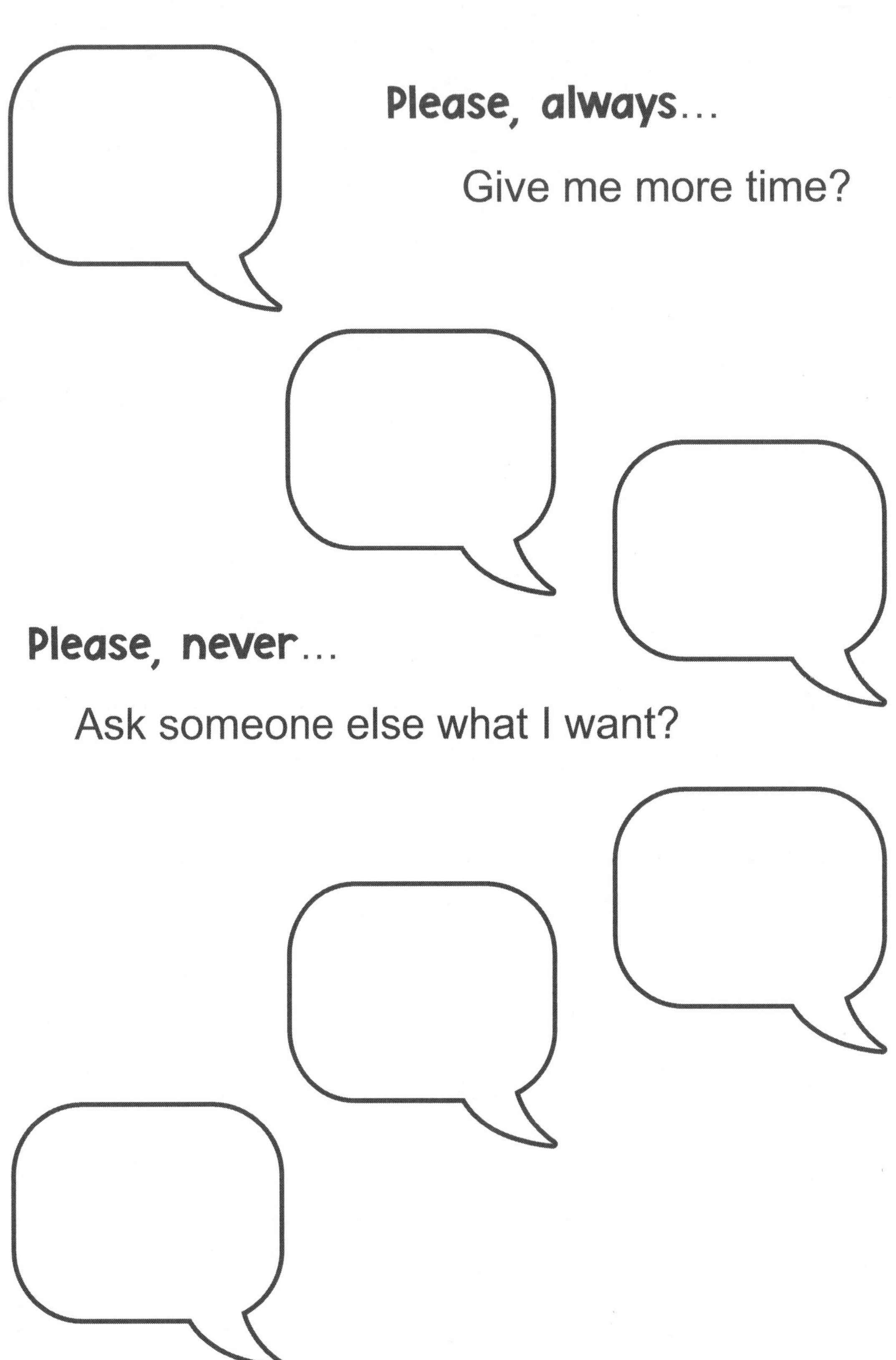

I want the world to know 

There need to be changes in: _______________________

____

____

____

People need to realise that: _______________________

____

____

____

I myself never realised: ___________________________

____

____

____

People can make a difference by: ___________________

____

____

____

Thinking about: what I've learned

I concentrate best when:

I'm always inspired by:

I'm working on:

I want my family to understand that:

Living well

I've learnt to: _______________________

____

____

____

A turning point has been: _______________

____

____

____

It really helped when: _________________

____

____

____

My greatest area of resilience is: _________

____

____

____

Thinking about: what works for me

	Yes	No	Should try!
Phone reminders?	☐	☐	☐
Checklists?	☐	☐	☐
Blogging or social media?	☐	☐	☐
Brain training?	☐	☐	☐
Exercise routine?	☐	☐	☐
Getting outside?	☐	☐	☐
Making things?	☐	☐	☐
Meditation?	☐	☐	☐
Naps?	☐	☐	☐
_________________	☐	☐	☐
_________________	☐	☐	☐
_________________	☐	☐	☐

My strategies

I am determined to: ________________________

____

____

I'm willing to accept help with: ______________

____

____

If I get tired, I need to: ___________________

____

____

Every day, I need to: _______________________

____

____

Thinking about: advice I'd give

t

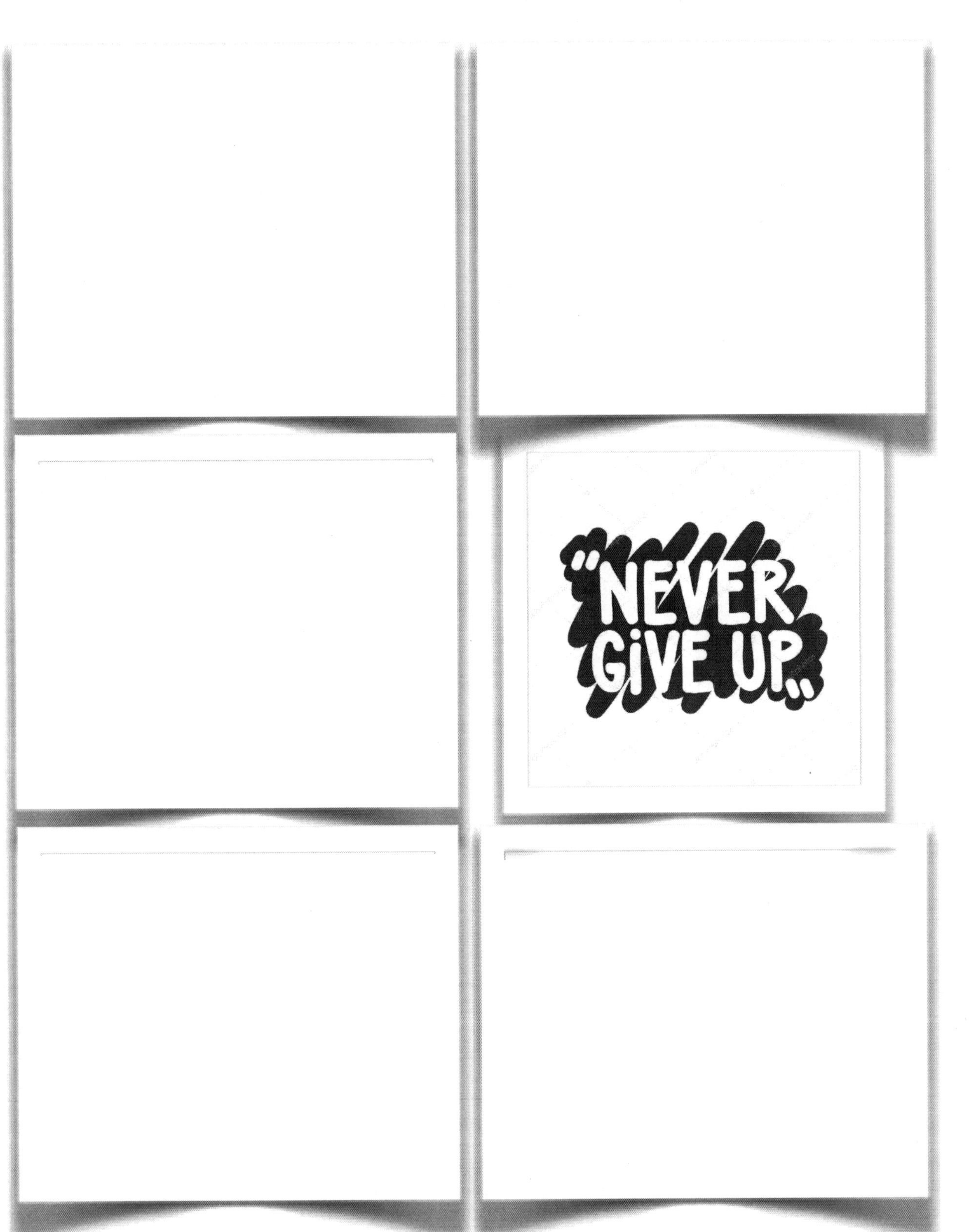

Wisdom and advice 

Advice I'd share with kids today: _______________

____

____

____

My philosophy of life is: _______________________

____

____

____

Thoughts for anyone facing challenges: _______________

____

____

____

Things it took me time to learn: _______________

____

____

____

Thinking about: instant lifts

Videos of baby elephants? 

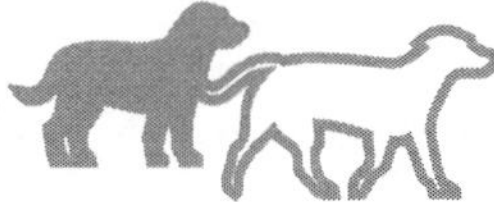 Sitting near a dog park?

World Cup highlights?

Singing along to 1980s hits?

Planting, weeding?

My 5 top instant lifts:

____

____

____

____

____

Simple pleasures 

It's a real buzz when: _______________________

____

____

I really must do more: _______________________

____

____

I like 'giving back' by: _______________________

____

____

I like to celebrate: _______________________

____

____

Thinking about: what's next?

Have fun by:

Make a difference by:

Appreciate life by:

Create something by:

What I want now

The most important thing in my life is: ___________

____

____

I'd really like to: ___________

____

____

I want to make a difference by: ___________

____

____

I'm lucky to: ___________

____

____

More about

More about

More about

More about

More about

____

More about

____

More about

____

More about

More about

More about

More about

More about

Congratulations

Congratulations
on taking the time to record
your story and your reflections.

This is valuable work, for you
and for the people around you.

Only you can tell your story.
Your experience is unique.

If you enjoyed using this book, please
consider leaving a review, or making
suggestions for future unforgettable books!

Thanks to Deposit Photos: incomible, hendry85, lhfgraphics, kharlmova_lv, Aluna11, vectorstank, pyty, Vanzyst

Made in the USA
Monee, IL
07 July 2026

56548202R00061